STOP the PAIN

Advance Praise

"*Stop the Pain* captured my imagination and I read it straight through in one sitting. I had a burning pain between my neck and shoulder before I started reading and was able to apply the release technique and the pain went away! Thank you!"

–**Marge D.**, in Kansas

"This is a completely different result than what my doctor told me—which was that my arm might hurt for the rest of my life after I hurt it in a fall. To make it feel better, I was doing everything wrong. I thought, 'no pain, no gain' and 'feel the burn.' Instead this expert has you focus on comfort and tune in to your body's signals. My arm is a thousand times better. I'm honestly amazed."

–**Jacqueline D.**, in Kansas

"As a young athlete, I always had a relationship with pain. Injury and muscle soreness were a common occurrence. I always had the "tough it out" mentality, fighting through pain, not listening to the messages my body was sending me. It wasn't until later in life that I realized the importance of rest and recovery in order to achieve my goal of longevity in my martial arts career. I always thought moving towards pain was the answer to relief. It wasn't until working with Vienna and the methods she was developing that I discovered quite the opposite and developed a new relationship with pain and changed my relationship with my body forever."

—**Nathanael G.**, in Kansas

"This is a do-it-yourself fix for pain that most doctors can't understand and can't fix. I work in the medical/alternative health field, and I have been looking for answers to my pain for years, and this is new information to me that worked. Best of all, it costs less than a doctor's visit copay."

—**Susan K.**, in Colorado

"A thoughtful read with practical advice about how to obtain healing. The principles are easy to understand and implement due to the step-by-step guidance, diagrams, and referrals to instructional videos."

—**Rujeko M.**, in Washington, D.C.

"Reading this delightful book was like opening a gift box full of inspiration applicable in so many realms of life and pain. This easily read book provides captivating, practical, transparent, real help!"

—**Pam C.**, in Colorado

"*Stop the Pain* is an excellent read! I loved how understandable and reader friendly this book is. Vienna is certainly an expert in her field, but she makes it easy to navigate and understand what is causing pain. The exercises in the book were extremely helpful and have given me a new perspective on creating and maintaining comfort."

—**BreAnn J.**, in Kansas

"Thank you, Vienna, for sharing your years of experience in helping others *Stop the Pain*. The techniques described in the book are easy to understand and should become second nature with a little practice. I had a sore spot in my neck that had been nagging me all day. I was able to release it in under a minute. I look forward to studying and sharing this guide with others who are ready to take ownership of their health with the power in their own hands. Thank you for making a difference with this wonderful guide."

—**Debbie H.**, in Kansas

"I thoroughly enjoyed reading this book. It was well researched but written in a simple style to make the concepts easily understood. I appreciated the impartation of hope in each page. I was able to try some of the pain releasing techniques while reading the book in an airport waiting area."

—**Marie L.**, in Kansas

STOP
the PAIN

Your Hands-On Manual *for*
Neck *and* Back Relief

Vienna Dunham Schmidt

NEW YORK

LONDON • NASHVILLE • MELBOURNE • VANCOUVER

STOP the PAIN
Your Hands-On Manual *for* Neck *and* Back Relief

Published in New York, New York, by Morgan James Publishing in partnership with Difference Press. Morgan James is a trademark of Morgan James, LLC. www.MorganJamesPublishing.com

ISBN 978-1-64279-676-6 paperback
ISBN 978-1-64279-677-3 eBook
ISBN 978-1-64279-678-0 audio
Library of Congress Control Number: 2019907439

Cover Design: Jennifer Stimson
Editing: Todd Hunter, Jenn Bailey, and Ronda Wohl
Illustration Model: Jubilee Schmidt
Illustration Photos: Malakki Matters
Author Photo: Jubilee Schmidt

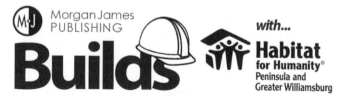

Morgan James is a proud partner of Habitat for Humanity Peninsula and Greater Williamsburg. Partners in building since 2006.

Get involved today! Visit
www.MorganJamesBuilds.com

DISCLAIMER

The author does not assume any responsibility for errors, omissions, or contrary interpretations of the subject matter herein. Any perceived slight of any individual or organization is purely unintentional.

Brand and product names are trademarks or registered trademarks of their respective owners.

Throughout this book the author has used examples from many of her clients' personal lives. However, to ensure privacy and confidentiality she has changed their names and some of the details of their experience. All the personal examples of the author's own life have not been altered.

The therapeutic information in this book is provided as an information resource only and is not to be used or relied on for any diagnostic or treatment purposes. This information is not intended to be patient education, does not create any patient-healthcare provider relationship, and should not be used as a substitute for professional diagnosis and treatment. Your healthcare provider can help you rule out the possibility of underlying disease and modify the contents of the book to meet your individual needs.

This handbook is dedicated to each of you who has shared your story, listened to my ideas about how to increase your comfort level, implemented them, and given valuable feedback. Believe me, I couldn't have done it without you!

TABLE OF CONTENTS

FOREWORD

This uncomplicated book invites readers to find a delightful oasis of attainable comfort. It grants readers a respite from a world of noise, clamor, busyness, pain, and strife. I love the threads of wisdom Vienna has woven through the instruction of this book. While those threads primarily apply to the relief of back, neck, and rib pain, they could be equally effective in many other areas of life. Even if you don't suffer from chronic pain and may be purchasing this book for a friend, please don't miss the opportunity to delve into this easy read for some golden nuggets you may apply in your own life! If you are one suffering with chronic pain, may you find answers and comfort here. This book will remind you that you are not alone, and there is definitely hope.

Over the two decades I have known Vienna as a friend, co-soccer mom, and massage therapist, she has consistently provided creative solutions to my own pain. She has honed her skills and developed a unique approach to an often-overlooked problem. What doctors and chiropractors may miss, her intuitive intelligence and persistent search for solutions has found. Vienna's approach is at once simple and straightforward, yet effective and profound.

As a wellness coach and counselor myself, I see strong parallels between our approaches to wellness. Having a rib out of place and dealing with the constant background noise of imbalance and pain can bleed imbalance into other areas of our lives. I love Vienna's healing paradigm of "going to the place of comfort," and have witnessed its effectiveness. This is definitely a cutting-edge idea and Vienna has a new message for those wanting to come into alignment, relieve pain, and dream again!

—**Pamela Christensen**, Boulder, Colorado

INTRODUCTION

"Change happens when the pain of staying the same is greater than the pain of change."
– Tony Robbins

The Perfect Storm of Chronic Pain

Since you are reading this book, you are probably acquainted with back pain or know someone who is. You are not alone. According to the American Chiropractic Association website, back pain is the most common cause of disability worldwide, and eight out of ten people in the United States will experience back pain at some point in their lives. For some, it's a brief encounter followed by occasional relapses. For others, it is a lifetime of never-ending consuming pain that defies description. Even though most of us fall somewhere in between, when pain lingers long enough, it can feel like it will never end. Perhaps it was a "perfect storm" of stressful events and strain on the body that brought it on, and the waves just seem to keep coming. The stress and tension created by chronic pain feed into each other until it is hard to remember what it is to feel fully relaxed. The impact is not confined to only our physical experience—it touches every aspect of our beings.

What If There Were a Choice?

We are familiar with chronic pain, but is there such a thing as "chronic comfort"? When negative experiences are shouting, it's easy to lose sight of the quieter places. Cultivating an attitude of gratitude for what is going well in the body will help us avoid taking areas of wellbeing for granted. Just as ongoing pain feels like dark clouds closing in around us, the seed of hope of the possibility of relief can be like the sun breaking through after a storm. Whether you've been enduring pain for thirty days or thirty years, the purpose and intent of this book is to model how to transition from pain into comfort. You will read and may watch in accompanying videos some strategies to help resolve your current distress and tension by using proven tools to achieve and maintain that comfort. By releasing tension in a way that doesn't cause discomfort, your body will begin to transition from a "fight, flight, or freeze" stress mode to a "rest and digest" peace mode. Even if the cause of your trouble goes beyond muscle tension (i.e., due to inflammation, injury, a pinched nerve, etc.), the presence of these types of pain can lead to increased tension, which in turn can amplify pain. The great news about this affordable self-care approach is that you are in control of when, where, and how much you use it. These pain-free techniques create positive side effects in the process of addressing the root causes of tension and pain.

Would you like to take a few minutes right now to close your eyes and think about what life will be like when your pain begins to give way to comfort? Imagine the sun coming out, the birds singing, and a soft, warm breeze blowing. Record that scene in your mind and heart and replay it often. I wish you peace, hope, and the start of a new chapter in your life!

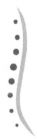

Chapter 1
YOUR PAIN IS REAL

"My pain is invisible. So is the pain you inflict when you don't believe me."
– ***Fibromyalgia News Today***, October 20, 2016

Sharon's Story

Sharon called and introduced herself on a Wednesday morning and asked with a tentative voice, as if barely daring to hope, whether I might have time to do some bodywork for her that day. She had driven from her home three hours away for an appointment with Linda, the clinical thermographer I used to work with. During the appointment with Linda, Sharon mentioned a long-term stabbing pain by her shoulder blade that had flared up during her drive. Linda, who had experienced a similar problem and gotten relief when had done bodywork with her, pointed Sharon in my direction. Thankfully, I had an opening right away.

I could read the stress on Sharon's face and hear the desperation in her voice as she described fifteen years of pain in her upper back and the various measures she had tried for relief. Sharon had been a stay-at-home mom, but the ever-present stabbing sensations prevented her from enjoying many activities with her two sons. As time went by, other chronic health challenges arose that pulled her down further. After her sons left for college, she had a desire to go back to school and gain new skills to enter the work force. The roller coaster of bad days and worse days with her back and health issues made her feel that her dream was too challenging to accomplish.

Sharon had started her quest for relief from back pain several years ago with her family doctor. She was referred to a specialist who ran various tests and then sent her to physical therapy. Physical therapy was an agonizing experience and the exercises for home use weren't helping. Through the years, there were more doctors, chiropractors, massage therapists, physical therapists, acupuncturists, medications, psychotherapy, and counselors. She recalled being dismissed from care on three occasions because the provider had nothing further to offer, which was honest on their part but discouraging to her.

Sometimes massage therapy would provide some relief for a few days, but it was not a complete or lasting solution. One therapist suggested she try some trigger point therapy at home on the most painful spot between her shoulder blades by rolling on a baseball. Even with repeated attempts with this therapy, her suffering increased rather than decreased. It was striking to me that she had been so committed to finding a solution that she was willing to try that harsh advice more than once!

As anyone knows who has tried various therapies long-term looking for relief, the expenses can add up, especially for alternative therapies that insurance does not cover. The atmosphere of financial stress can lead to tension in relationships. Eventually hopelessness can move in as a companion to chronic pain. For Sharon, these stresses compounded and created the terrifying, desperate, and out-of-control sensation of a downward spiral.

From her description of the stabbing pain between her shoulder blade and spine, I suspected that one or more ribs had been pushed or pulled out of their ideal position. A quick check confirmed this. I applied the muscle release techniques (see chapter 5) and she began to feel relief. As we worked together over the next hour, her stated pain level went from ten to zero on a ten-point scale.

Since she lived a few hours away and it was uncertain when we could get together again, I made a persuasive case for the necessity of self-care. We made a ten-minute video on her phone to remind her of the home care version of the techniques, and she headed back home. When I checked in with her later, Sharon reported that she was using the short video reminder daily to move forward in releasing muscle tension. The relief from our session lasted several days until she did some awkward lifting that aggravated the area. She did the home care procedures and got the pain from an eight on the scale to a two in about twenty minutes. She felt empowered because she could re-create the relief for herself at home. The next step was to do a video call and consider what factors in her daily life were causing the tension that put strain on the ribs. By thinking consciously about her environment and activities, Sharon can make adjustments and avoid reinjury.

I was very excited to watch Sharon as she experienced increased comfort and the hope that she could regain her health and sense of wellbeing and move forward toward her dreams. I believe the principles and activities in this book can make a difference for you too as you apply them to your areas of muscle tension and pain.

Your New Chapter

I want to validate that your pain is real. Having people not understand that you are going through difficult things is hard; having them not believe you at all is even worse. A part of the frustration for many people who suffer with chronic pain is the experience of having a medical authority state that they can't find anything wrong. Whether from an outside source or an internal voice, it is possible to interpret that message as, "It's all in your head." I have had clients share that they felt like exploding when a doctor referred them for a psychological evaluation because the cause of their suffering was invisible. If you are exhausted from trying to find answers to your chronic pain questions, I invite you to see if the strategies presented in these pages provide a way for you to bring relief with your own hands.

Since you are the only one who knows what you feel, I believe you are uniquely qualified to take the steps to release the chronic tension and pain that have been like a shadow eclipsing your comfort. I firmly believe that you can make a difference for yourself and reduce or eliminate your distress and that this is the perfect time for you to experience a shift toward comfort.

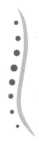

Chapter 2
THERE IS A WAY OUT

"Healing is a matter of time, but it is also sometimes a matter of opportunity."

– Hippocrates

Why It Matters to Me

I first observed the beneficial effects of massage at home in my teen years. My youngest brother suffered from severe neck tension as an infant that may have been a result of his delivery with forceps. He would writhe and cry in pain, his head drawing to one side. It amazed me how my Dad could quiet him by rubbing his neck. Soon my brother's neck would straighten, and he would smile. When I was a teenager, I did my first bodywork, massaging my Dad's shoulder for bursitis pain. I was amazed and glad that some simple hand movements could bring him relief.

My journey toward understanding the startlingly simple strategies in this book included working in my family's veterinary clinic from the age of twelve. The scientific atmosphere fed my natural interest in how things work and why they happen, especially with living things. I am a persistent and patient person by nature and don't mind spending several hours at a time researching and problem solving.

I gained empathy for those experiencing back pain from my experience with mild scoliosis, which was detected by a chiropractor in my early teen years. I am grateful that the pain was never debilitating. My pain would flare up, first during high school and college because of long hours of studying, and later, while I was pregnant and caring for my young children. I found intermittent relief with consistent chiropractic care, though spasms would sometimes wake me after a few hours of sleep if I aggravated my back during the day.

During college, I desperately wanted to know my purpose in life, asking, "Where is my niche?" Often at 10:00 p.m., when the library closed, a line would form at my dorm door consisting of people with neck and upper back pain. I was puzzled why no one else was helping them, as it seemed to me that anyone could do this bodywork. Now I find it amusing that I was begging to know my destiny and totally missing the answer right at my fingertips!

Wherever I went through the years, I helped friends and family with their pain. It wasn't until I was in my early forties that I recognized that what I was doing with my hands was the gift I was longing to find.

My New Chapter

In 2003, I had a backyard neighbor, Beverly, whom I saw weekly at church, but did not talk with or see often otherwise. One day, when I happened to call to ask a question, she sounded distraught. She said she had severe neck pain and had not slept much in five days, so I offered to come over and rub her neck a bit. After about an hour of using calming strokes and gentle pressure on the tense muscles, the pain was gone. She had movement in her neck again. She asked how much I would charge to come regularly, and she became my most consistent customer and my biggest promoter by giving bodywork gift certificates to friends and family. When I saw myself being consistently energized by this work, I realized I had finally found my gift!

I continued helping those close to me when a need arose and then a chiropractor introduced me to a painless and very effective muscle release technique called Ortho-Bionomy. I eagerly took an introductory level course, and the principles I learned in that class are at the heart of some of the release techniques that I share in this manual. I next took a training program to become a licensed massage therapist. One of the unexpected benefits of getting regular massages during the training program, combined with regular chiropractic care at Cleveland University, was a significant improvement in my scoliosis. My back is the happiest I can remember it being. Even if I aggravate my back or neck, the strategies in the following chapters have brought me consistent and welcome relief.

As I gained experience, I began to see patterns of chronic pain in my clients, so I put my curiosity and problem-solving abilities to work. I found that a variety of muscle release techniques were the most effective tools I had learned, but

I struggled with finding a way to reassure my clients that work was being done during the thirty-second hold that is part of the muscle release process. Clients came in with the expectation of a traditional massage—one of continuous fluid movements—and I was holding muscles still. I had only recently graduated from massage school and was lacking confidence in the delivery of my skills.

I breathed a prayer for help and a little story started to flow through me. The story kept the client's mind occupied while I held the release position. After feeling the profound and painless release, clients were usually very willing to continue on that path. With each client, the story developed, phrase-by-phrase, narrating the way the body can end up in a seemingly endless loop of pain and tension and then find relief through comfort and ease. I share this entertaining parable with you in the next chapter.

Now I get to wake up every day and live my dream of helping people find their way out of pain and into freedom through bodywork. I love sharing an individualized form of the training in this manual so they can practice self-care at home to maintain the results we see in sessions, even when facing the stresses of daily life. I am sharing the same information with you here, and in the videos on my website, to make it easy for you to follow the techniques and find relief for yourself!

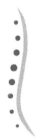

Chapter 3

HOME WHERE
I BELONG

"Well-being or wholeness implies integrity and harmony between all existing elements, providing freedom for the whole."

– Darrell Calkins

Once Upon a Time

Every part of your body has a home, and in that home, there's a comfortable chair where it really likes to sit. This includes every bone, muscle, tendon, ligament, nerve, and blood vessel—everything! Before you were born, each part of you was in its comfy chair. After your birth, through the bumps and bruises of life, maybe after an accident or two, some of your parts have probably come out of their comfy chair—maybe even out of their home. You might find one in the backyard…in the rain…crying!

Well, when the neighboring parts hear the commotion, they come running. "Is everything OK out there?"

"No, I hurt!"

"We'll stand with you, until help comes." those neighboring parts say.

That is, after all, the neighborly thing to do. But it makes things tense, because now nobody is in their comfy chair. And if it goes on long enough, those neighbors might call to their neighbors, who might call to their neighbors, and your little problem grows into a much bigger problem.

One thing that's true of these tight muscles is that they are wrung-out muscles with very little blood flow. And without blood flow, you know what they're missing—oxygen, nutrients, and somebody to come by and take out the trash. So toxins start piling up, which causes other problems. This neighborhood needs more blood flow as soon as possible!

There are several ways to help this happen. One is to add heat to the area. You can tell heat is increasing blood flow because the area becomes red. However, that only helps the top few centimeters of the tissue. For deeper tension, we need to find an additional strategy. Some other possibilities to increase blood flow are pressure, vibration, tapping, and other kinds of action that stimulate the tissue.

Often, people will turn to stretch to help loosen up a tight muscle. But a sudden deep stretch can create a fear response and the muscle may lock down even tighter to protect itself. A gentle stretch on a warmed-up muscle can help bring in more blood flow as you begin to release the stretch. In my experience, a stretch can bring in enough blood flow for a muscle to get inside the back door again, but it needs have even more blood coming in to help it be completely pliable to reach all the way to its comfy chair.

One of the most effective ways I've found to bring in maximum blood flow is to put a muscle at rest. When a muscle is slack, there is more space for more blood to come in, so the muscle can fill more completely, which allows it to reach all the way to its comfy chair.

I like to compare it to a damp sponge that you squeeze in your fist. If you put your hand in a bucket of water, but don't let go of the sponge, nothing changes. But if you do let go, the sponge fills completely—and quickly. Why? Because it can. If there is space, it will fill.

When a muscle is put at rest (or made slack) for twenty to forty-five seconds, it fills with blood effortlessly as your heart is circulating blood throughout your body. Once full, it can't be that tight, wrung-out muscle anymore. Giving a little circular movement to the one that was in the backyard lets everyone in the neighborhood know, "I'm headed home now, and you can go home, too!"

Chapter 4 will show you how to apply the muscle release technique described in the story to your body for relief of pain and tension. You can hear the story in the video **"Home Where I Belong"** on the website below.

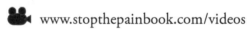 www.stopthepainbook.com/videos

A Paradigm Shift: Lean into Comfort

What is a paradigm shift? Merriam-Webster defines it as, "an important change that happens when the usual way of thinking about or doing something is replaced by a new and different way."

A current example of a paradigm shift in medical understanding is based on SPECT brain scan technology popularized by Dr. Daniel Amen. He notes that we used to think we were stuck with the brain we were born with.

Today, with this imaging, we can clearly see the impact that our diet, exercise, sleep, and a myriad of other factors have on our brains. Our brains are capable of surprising levels of development and repair (Dr. Amen on TedX). This concept of neuroplasticity is now widely accepted and has revolutionized the way we think about brain health. This example of a paradigm shift in understanding has brought hope to people with head injuries, dementia, addictions, and other brain-related ailments.

Regarding the topic of pain, especially as it relates to muscle tension, one element of our current paradigm or mindset in the United States is often stated as, "No pain, no gain!" To watch people cringing while they roll out tight muscles with a foam roller at the gym or demanding an ever-increasing amount of pressure during a massage, it would seem that they also believe that, "Pain *is* gain," and that increased discomfort and pressure will somehow result in relief for their pain or tension. Part of the purpose of pain in the big picture of our lives is to wave a red flag to alert us that something is wrong so that we will pay attention, move away from what is causing the pain, and take steps to solve the problem.

You are the insider in your body, so only you can know how your body is responding to painful stimuli. I encourage you to check in with what your body is feeling when your activity is causing pain to see if the net result is release or tension. Generally speaking, in the presence of pain, the sympathetic nervous system is stimulated to release stress hormones, which tell the body to run away, freeze, or fight against what is happening. In the presence of the stress hormones, tension and pain can escalate.

With the pain free bodywork you are learning in this book, the parasympathetic nervous system is activated, and the hormones that calm the body and release tension begin to circulate with the message of "rest and digest." One of my co-workers says of the concept of pain-free muscle release techniques: "No pain, all gain!" By moving a muscle in the direction of comfort (away from pain), we are setting it up to fill with blood and be able to be pliable enough to reach all the way back to its comfy chair. When its neighbors get the message, they head home too, and the neighborhood becomes a peaceful, balanced place. Clients are often shocked by the simplicity and gentleness of these techniques and relieved to find that comfort was so close at hand. I am grateful to have found a great deal of gain in comfortable muscle release for both my clients and me.

I encourage you to make the paradigm shift to lean into comfort rather than pain. In the introduction to *Ortho-Bionomy: A Path to Self-Care*, Luann Overmyer speaks of the release technique as providing "a new way to think about pain and restriction that creates permanent, positive change." Ortho-bionomy concepts have influenced the muscle release techniques described in chapters 4 and 5.

Since I have started thinking in terms of relaxation and release for muscles in the physical realm, I have seen parallels in other areas of life and now notice other people expressing the concept of leaning into rest in different contexts. For example, Andy Puddicombe's app for mindfulness called *Headspace* has a lesson regarding creative thought. He explains that "trying hard" to control our thoughts and press them into focus is actually an unproductive strategy because it creates restrictions in our thinking. His suggestion is to release our grip on our mind and thoughts and simply notice, without judgement, what is going on in our thinking. This way we can restore the flow of ideas and creativity. With regard to our heart and soul, it is widely held that if we hold on to pain or offences, a restriction of flow is created. By choosing to forgive and release our hold on negative emotions, flow can be restored and bring with it positive emotions and freedom.

Finding release and flow is highly beneficial. For example, I had an interview I was nervous about, and I experienced a shutdown of both thinking and feeling. My life coach encouraged me to look for the place of flow in my heart where I could be authentic in order to get out of the corner of fear I had backed myself into. After taking her advice to talk about the work I love, my peace and ability to think returned immediately. As a result, I was calm and focused during the phone interview and I was accepted into the program I was applying to.

I have also seen this idea work in the delicate balance of the hormones and chemicals in the body. If this area is of interest to you, an increasing amount of information is available in books and websites like *The Adrenal Fatigue Solution* by Fawne Hansen and *Silent Takeover: How the Body Hijacks the Mind* by Jacquelyn Sheppard. They provide insight about the key role of bringing our nervous systems back into balance to reduce muscle tension.

Another key principle in release techniques is that muscle tension and blood flow are inversely proportional, so when tension comes in, blood is squeezed out. When blood flow is returned (in this case, by making a muscle slack), tension must leave. The pain and tension cycle in the body can be seen as a spiral. When tension comes in and blood goes out of a muscle, a nearby bone may be shifted slightly out of position, a nerve may be squeezed, other neighboring parts may spring from their chairs, and pain can result. In response to the pain, the muscle may tighten even more, and the cycle continues until more neighbors get involved and larger movements are restricted. This would be a negative spiral.

The cycle can be interrupted and reversed at any point. You can change the direction of movement from pain toward comfort and relaxation. For example, heat can be applied to allow some blood to come in, which means some tension goes out and the area is more comfortable and relaxed. Some ways that heat can be applied are a heated rice bag, hot water bottle, heating pad, hot bath or shower, aromatherapy pillow, or hot stone massage. Check with your healthcare provider about whether heat or cool is more appropriate for your particular discomfort. Generally speaking, heat is not suggested for a new injury or an inflamed area.

To further unwind the tension, you can add another strategy, like doing some mindful breathing, which reduces the stress hormones and prompts the muscles to begin to relax and allow more blood to come in. There are many apps available now that encourage and train users in effective breathing and the art of mindfulness. You might want to try a few of them to find one that resonates.

When we know some of the events that may introduce tension to the body, we can take steps to correct or prevent them from happening. An emergency (whether perceived or real) produces tension throughout the body. When we trip, the instantaneous reaction of contraction is an effort to rescue us from falling. Whether or not we actually fall (as long as there is not a severe injury) most of the body will get the memo that the emergency is over, allowing the muscles to relax, and blood flow to return. However, a few muscles may not get the message and may remain tight, which will set off the chain reaction of decreased blood flow mentioned earlier. Being aware of the tension enables you to take steps to release it and restore balance to your body and its movements.

Other examples of potential stressors on the body include being cold (shivering), rush hour traffic, an argument, a deadline, an exam, expectations, or lack of sleep. The strategies mentioned above and some in later chapters may help the body get to a more peaceful place. Surgery is also interpreted as an emergency in the body and muscles around the incision may not get the message that the emergency is over. Those muscles may need to have the message delivered by hand with some of the muscle release techniques detailed in the following chapters.

When a person is in chronic pain that has no obvious physical cause, they can feel very frustrated, disregarded, and alone. It may even be suggested that the pain is all in their head, so to speak. This book is about releasing muscle tension that causes very real pain, whether the source of the tension is physical, mental, or emotional. In chapter 6 there are some references to strategies that may help release overall stress. Stress of any kind takes a tremendous toll on the body, and western culture is just beginning to understand the mind/body connection at a deeper level.

Dr. Thomas Holmes and Dr. Richard Rahe, both psychiatrists, put together a list of life experiences, both positive and negative, that have been found to impact people and illustrate the toll that the stress of change can have in people's lives. For example, losing a job is an obvious stressor, but getting a raise also requires adjustments and creates stress. An online version of the *Life Stress Assessment* can be found on the American Institute of Stress website at www.stress.org/holmes-rahe-stress-inventory.

Knowing that an event has the potential to produce a stress response is a first step toward reducing its effects. If you are feeling isolated or alone in your pain, consider sharing the results of the assessment with a friend or counselor, which can also keep you moving on the journey toward releasing tension in your muscles, as well as other deeper levels of your being. If you are interested in learning more about the connection between the brain and the body specifically as it relates to chronic pain and healing, Rick Olderman gives some helpful details in *Fixing You: Back Pain*.

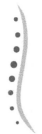

Chapter 4
WHAT HAVE YOU GOT TO LOSE BUT YOUR PAIN?

"Knowledge isn't power until it's applied."
– Dale Carnegie

Preparing to Trade Pain for Comfort

It is my firm belief that the ideas and actions you will apply as you read this chapter have the potential to change your life. In your busy world distractions may come up as you are reading. I encourage you to let them go by and focus on this process for the next thirty minutes so that you can practice what you are learning and start your journey out of pain right now. You can also follow along with the **"Muscle Release Overview"** video from the following webpage.

🎥 **Video:** www.stopthepainbook.com/videos

For the "Note" step below, have a pen and paper handy to take notes about the sensations you notice in your body. If you prefer to record what you observe visually or in more detail, you can do an Internet search for "medical body image" and print out a blank body form on which you can draw your observations. As you prepare for the "Release" phase, it is important to notice where pain is in your body so you can decide where to begin to apply these simple techniques.

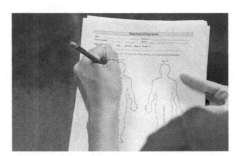

Fig. 1. Medical body image for notes, optional

I hope the following instructions can make this potentially transformative method seem alive and easy for you. The flowchart below gives an overview of the process to refer back to once you have read through the detailed instructions. Watching the **"Muscle Release Flowchart"** video may also be helpful.

Video: www.stopthepainbook.com/videos

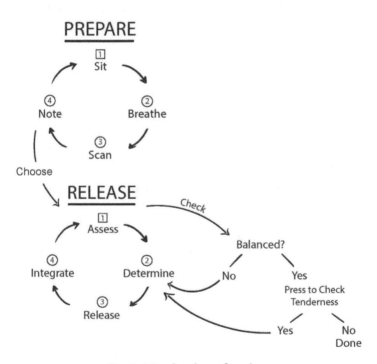

Fig. 2. Muscle release flowchart

The Road Home

I recommend watching the **"Muscle Release Technique"** video before you begin in order to make the instructions easier to follow.

 Video: www.stopthepainbook.com/videos

Preparation Phase

P1. Sit: Take a few moments to get comfortable in a chair that is firm enough that you won't sink into it, which can restrict your movements. Have your pen and paper nearby.

P2. Breathe: Take a few breaths, releasing tension as you exhale. Notice how the breath feels going in through your nose and out through your mouth. (This type of breathing is not about how deeply you breathe, but about being focused or mindful as you breathe. Don't worry about trying to "get it right," just try to let go of any restriction in your breathing.)

P3. Scan: Now turn your focus from your breathing to your body. Close your eyes and slowly notice each part of your body. Start at the top of your head. Move to your jaw and face. Is there tension in your neck? Is it more on one side than the other? Now notice your upper back and shoulders. Then think about your hands and arms. Move on down to your mid-back and ribs. Take a few deeper breaths to expand your ribs; do you notice any discomfort or restriction in any area of the ribs. Now move on to your abdomen and pay attention to any sensations there. Is there any discomfort in your low back or hips?

Slowly move your attention down your legs to your knees. Notice how your feet are feeling. Is there any tension, discomfort, or pain? (The focus of this book is neck and back pain, but your body can't be persuaded to isolate one area from another, and each area is impacted by its neighbors both near and far. By noticing pain in every area, we open the possibility of finding connections of tension we were not aware of before. The release technique works on any area of the body.)

P4. Note: Did you find discomfort, pain, or tension? Make a list on paper or mark it on a medical body image page (which can be printed from the internet). Include a number from the pain scale and any descriptive words. You can use a typical pain scale where 0 is no pain and 10 is the worst pain you can imagine. There is no right or wrong answer and it seems to get easier with practice. I believe using the number scale can make our observations more objective and helps us to notice changes.

One of the miracles of the human experience is the capacity we have to forget exactly what the pain felt like after it is gone. Descriptive words for pain include the following: sharp, stabbing, vice-like, gnawing, throbbing, dull, achy, tingling, burning, itching, numb, pins and needles, stinging, sensitive to touch, tender, sore, heavy congested, tight, irritated, acute, chronic, cold, chilly, warm, feverish, hot, inflamed.

If you found several areas with pain, it's fine to mentally scan your body again. It is helpful to include each area that you notice on your list. If you have pain in so many areas that making a comprehensive list is overwhelming, don't worry about completing the list in one sitting. Just pick an area that is important to you for your first release. It's more important not to add stress in the process of releasing stress.

Choose: "Choose" is the action step between the "Prepare" and "Release" phases. You may want to select the area that is hurting the most. While you are learning the technique, pick an area with pain or tenderness that you can reach easily. Mid-back pain or knots/stabbing pain between the shoulder blades will be addressed in the next chapter, so I recommend choosing a different area to learn the technique in this chapter.

Release Phase

Change your focus from noticing pain to observing where the sensation of comfort is during this Release phase. There are four reasons I encourage you to notice where comfort is and move toward it.

1. Remember the sponge analogy from the story in the last chapter? The goal is to allow the tense muscles to fill with blood by making them slack. Blood flow and tension can be seen as inversely proportional—when tension comes in, blood flow goes out. And when blood flow is allowed in, tension must go out to the same degree. Without blood flow the muscle cells are starved of oxygen and nutrients, and they lose the capacity to get rid of toxins.

2. Where we focus our attention is important. When I'm walking down a sidewalk, I focus my attention on the direction I wish to go. I face toward my goal. I believe that your intention in reading this book is to arrive at a place of comfort, so all release activities are done with comfort in mind.

3. Pain is a red flag waving in the body to say that something is wrong. The muscle release method is

designed to be a completely comfortable and safe way to release tension, so there is no need to press through the red flag of pain to find comfort.

4. Pain causes the body to respond with stress hormones and the stimulation of the sympathetic nervous system, characterized by "fight, flight, or freeze." It is beneficial to move toward comfort, where the parasympathetic nervous system is awakened, and the hormones are released that lead to "rest and digest."

R1. Assess: Put two fingers gently on top of the sore or tender place you chose to release and press in lightly to see what number on the pain scale (0-10) you would give the discomfort. Write the number down next to the pain scale number you gave the area during the Scan step. Also make a note of any additional descriptive words that come to mind.

R2. Determine:

This important step guides the release that brings relief in the next step.

1. Place two fingers lightly on the sore area again with just enough pressure to move the muscle a bit

without your fingers sliding across the skin. Use the amount of pressure you might use to see if a piece of fruit is soft and ripe. If that is too sore, use lighter pressure.

2. Keeping your fingers together, move them in two opposing directions, like upward and downward, or left and right. Think of it as more of a press than a push.

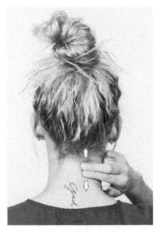

Fig. 3. Example of muscle release position on neck

3. Determine how the two opposite directions feel.
   o They feel the same, both hurt
   o They feel the same, both are comfortable

o There is a difference between them. One direction is more comfortable and has more ease of movement than the other.

You are specifically looking for the line of movement that has a difference between the two opposite muscles. This difference points to an imbalance that can be corrected by moving toward comfort. Comfort puts the area of tension at rest so it can fill with blood and bring balance to the area.

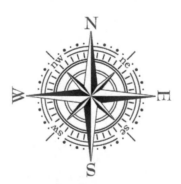

Fig. 4. Compass to illustrate potential release positions

There are attachments in all directions on every part of your body, which can be compared to a compass to illustrate that you can have tension from any direction of the 360 degrees around the central point of pain. The four primary compass directions (north, south, east, and west) and four secondary compass directions (northeast, southeast, northwest, southwest) usually cover the whole area, as far as releasing tension. The direction itself and the order that you check them in is not important. What matters is finding and releasing opposite directions that are out of balance.

Even when a spot is very tense or tender, usually one or more of the eight directions of release will be comfortable or at least bearable. On the rare occasion that all the eight directions are very uncomfortable, you can press in on the muscle lightly and move or lightly twist the tissue under your fingers in a clockwise and counterclockwise direction to see if one of those opposite directions is comfortable.

R3. Release: Hold gently in the direction of comfort for twenty to forty-five seconds. This hold is an invitation to feel and sense flow, not to force in an effort to cause something to happen. Less holding time may be needed if there is less tension initially because the muscle is not as wrung out, in terms of blood flow.

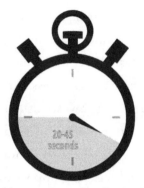

Fig. 5. Hold toward comfort for 20-45 seconds

R4. Integrate: At the end of the release move, make a few small circles with your fingers in either direction to get everyone on the same page. It serves as a notice of the change of address that lets the neighbors know the muscle you were working with has headed home, and they can, too.

Check: See if the two opposite directions you checked before feel similar or "balanced" now, like both muscles are equally relaxed. If they are, one full cycle is completed. Areas with low to moderate tension may only need one cycle to get every body part home and in their comfy chair. By repeating the Assess step, you can determine whether there is still tenderness suggesting you need do another cycle.

Reassess: If the answer to the Assess step question, "Is there tenderness?" is now "No," you can check nearby areas for tenderness on which to begin the cycle or go to the next area on the list.

If the answer to the Assess step is still "Yes," rate the remaining tenderness you found, and repeat the Release step.

Release: The spot may need one more round in the same direction, or it may be ready to release tension in the opposite direction. Your body will indicate what it needs; all you need to do is move the tissue under your fingers in the direction of ease and comfort. Go through the full cycle again, which takes less than a minute.

When the body indicates that it is ready to go in the opposite direction, it may seem like the pain has moved. In a situation such as this, I believe both areas of discomfort were there all along and the first sensation was like an alarm that was so loud that you couldn't even hear the second one until the first one was quiet.

If there is still tension or tenderness at the end of the second cycle, check the diagonal directions that make an X on the compass—northeast and southwest; northwest and southeast. (An area that is very sore may seem like it won't have any direction that is comfortable, but in my experience, there is usually at least one of the eight that is not tender or is quite a bit less tender than the others and that is the best place to start.)

Repeat the cycle until the Assess step has no tenderness. If you have released all eight compass directions and still find tenderness, the next step is to place two fingers on the tender spot again and hold the fingers together as you turn them slightly in a clockwise and then a counterclockwise direction. Again, if there is a difference, go in the direction of comfort and ease of movement. Hold twenty to forty-five seconds, do the integrative circle, and recheck. If you still have tenderness, let the area rest for a few minutes while you release another spot and come back to check it later.

If trying to follow the whole release process with words alone is challenging, I encourage you to go to the website and hear it with explanations in the Overview video. In the **"Guided Muscle Release"** video, you will be led through a sample process verbally so you don't need to be looking at the book.

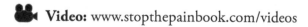 **Video:** www.stopthepainbook.com/videos

Sometimes after a release you might feel that a spot is much less tender, and feel ready to move on to the next area. I think of an incomplete release as "tolerable recovery." I know can be hard to imagine that the tenderness will go away completely, but typically it does when each part is in their comfy chair. I encourage you to try another round or two of the release sequence when there is even a slight bit of tenderness or tension remaining to see if the last little step to get to the comfy chair can be taken care of right then.

In the unusual event that there is still a strong pain or other sensation after you have watched the video and released the rest of the area, feel free to email me your experiences or questions at vienna@stopthepainbook.com. If it is difficult to put into written words, we can schedule a video conference call to see if it would make sense to work together to stop the pain. I have seen this release method work so well for so many people that I want to be sure that you have every opportunity to learn and implement it effectively for yourself.

Stay curious and aware of any sensation as blood flow comes in. Some people notice warmth and others feel a sensation like an area is tingling or coming alive again as nerve impulses and blood flow return. Don't worry if you don't notice anything. The area is definitely filling with blood, because you are creating space for it by putting the area at rest. When chronic pain has gone on for a while, all messages may be felt less acutely—both pain and comfort. As it becomes "safe" to listen to messages again as comfort increases, you may be able to tune in more easily to the good news messages of release and balance in your body.

When pain suddenly no longer exists in an area it is very tempting "look for the pain" or quickly put the area through its full range of motion to convince yourself that it's really better. I encourage you to be gentle with the area and make small movements first. Save the more vigorous test for twenty-four to forty-eight hours later so that all the body members involved can get used to being in their comfy chairs. People are often relieved when I tell them they shouldn't vacuum or rake leaves or shovel snow for a few days so things don't return to the old familiar out of place pattern before they've gotten used to being home again.

I made the mistake of ignoring this advice myself some time ago. I got some ribs back home after a fall and the area felt so good right away that I went and carried some heavy bags, which was not a good idea. It took me a few more days of intermittent effort to get them persuaded to go home again.

At first, it may seem impossible that it could be so simple to release tension and relieve pain. Here's how easy it is: I taught this technique to a five-year-old, and we released her areas of tension. The next morning, she came downstairs with the original pain completely gone. She told her mom that her elbow was hurting, which was a new pain. Then she remembered her new tool and said, "Wait, maybe it's not home." She followed the steps and within a minute, she reported, "Oh, never mind, it went home!"

How different would life be if we had all learned muscle tension release techniques in kindergarten? This young generation could have a very different experience with comfort if they have an opportunity to learn these principles early. All of us can have hope that we can have a fresh start now, at any age!

If a person has an area that has been sore for a long time, they may not remember the event that caused the tension and pain. For some, within a few minutes to hours of releasing the tension, the memory of the accident that happened will come to them "out of the blue." It seems that memories can be stored in the body itself and when the tension is released, the memory can also be released after a fairly short period of time.

One of the most striking examples was a client who had a few ribs very misaligned and had no memory of how that may have happened. It took about thirty minutes to release all the related tension, but the ribs finally settled back in their comfy chairs. She had no memory of any impacts or accidents, so I mentioned that the memory could come to her later. I also suggested that she might consider being attentive and kind to herself, as I felt it must surely have been a significant impact. In about ten minutes, while I was working somewhere else on her body, she looked startled and said, "Oh, my goodness, in the fourth grade, I was hit by a school bus and thrown twenty feet away into a yard." She went on to say that she felt at fault for the accident because she had run across the street to meet someone without looking. She had jumped up and convinced everyone that she was fine and perhaps stuffed away the memory and the pain to avoid criticism from herself or others.

The way we are made is amazing and complex. If you become aware of an emotion rising after releasing a tender spot, try acknowledging the sensation and thinking of it like an ocean wave or a cloud and letting it go by. If it was a traumatic event, try releasing any accompanying emotional or mental pain in the moment. Trust yourself. Tears may come and are a beneficial form of release and cleansing.

Plant Good Seed

To use a gardening analogy, we can plant the seeds of what we want to harvest: stress and pain, or peace and comfort. Stress and pain levels impact each other. Certainly, when I have less pain, I have less ambient stress. When I have less stress response, I also perceive pain less acutely. One of my children found dental visits to be stressful as a young child. At one visit, the pediatric dentist gave him numbing shots three times, but he could still feel everything that was happening. When I came home and did some research, I found some sources that indicated that high levels of adrenalin could make the numbing shot ineffective. I believe our bodies will always be appreciative of any steps we take and new habits we develop in order to decrease our stress response to the events of life.

You are the insider when it comes to your body and you are uniquely suited to recognize pain and comfort and make the corrections necessary to shift the focus toward comfort. I invite you to consider a few questions, such as whether responsibility for your comfort lies inside or outside of you. What can you control? What can an outsider control inside of anyone? If you can work with these ideas and techniques, you not only will have the opportunity to take responsibility for your own comfort, but for even bigger picture things like health and happiness. Another person is not able to be as vested as you are in your outcomes done your way.

For me, this has been a major paradigm shift. I invite you to consider where you are now and where you would like to be with regard to your wellbeing. If your current reality and your goal don't fully match, you can begin to make small shifts to get on course with where you want to go. If you would like some helpful information and creative ideas, I recommend Dr. Michelle Robin's book *Small Changes Big Shifts*. She discusses the Four Quadrants of Wellbeing: Mechanical, Chemical, Energetic, and Psychospritual.

When I shared the idea of a paradigm shift from a pain focus to a focus on comfort with my transition coach, she had an "Aha!" moment. She was reminded of a difficult time in her life after an auto accident a few years ago when she had to spend a few weeks in the hospital. The care team would conscientiously come in every hour to ask her to rate her pain, and it was intensely frustrating for her. Pain was a harsh reality in several areas of her body, and it was a challenging feat to find a way to distract herself from the constant emergency messages bombarding her brain. If the "How would you rate your pain right now?" question invaded a rare moment of peace, it served to intensify her frustration and the sensation of pain.

As we spoke, she envisioned how the experience could have been transformed if they had come in hourly and asked what they could do *right now* to make her more comfortable. There is obviously a required protocol to assess pain so it can be documented and addressed medically, but when that is the primary focus, it can perpetuate the release of stress hormones and keep a person in pain mode. Her thought was that there were many times when a warm blanket or a cup of hot tea would have felt good and increased her sense of wellbeing. The shift away from the sympathetic nervous system operating in "fight, flee, or freeze" and toward the parasympathetic nervous system of "rest and digest" would have encouraged rest and healing. I recently spoke with a nursing student and was encouraged to hear that her program was emphasizing comfort measures for patients in a comprehensive response the current crisis of pain medication addiction.

Every part of your body matters! Every part of your body needs your care!

Can you think of a time you were impatient or rude with a part of your body that wasn't working the way you thought it should? The first time I was confronted with this idea of body rudeness, I had asked a client what issues she wanted to work on that day. She responded, "this darn shoulder." Her comment made me pause for thought and I suggested that she needed to recognize how important the shoulder's part was in her whole-body picture. Surely her shoulder didn't choose this pain. I encouraged her to apologize to her shoulder for her critical attitude and to invite that shoulder to come back home. The session went well, and she was pleased when the shoulder was restored to full function.

One way to think of the goal of this method is: "One area at a time, everybody gets to go home, and let's work together to reduce overall life and body stress so they can stay there." I encourage you to remain calm, even if you feel a twinge of the old familiar pain again later. You know what to do now, and it will not be able to be as strong now. If you get into a place that you can't figure out how to release it, feel free to contact me at vienna@stopthepainbook.com.

What will this technique work on? Try it on everything. Since you are always gently going toward comfort in this method, you are not putting any part of your body at risk. My rule of thumb is, if you can reach it, you can release it. And if you can't quite reach a place in your back, you might try a tool like a TheraCane®, which is shaped like a letter J that is about 24" high with large marble shapes in several locations. The ball on the hooked end can be placed on a tender spot on the back and slight pressure can be applied toward comfort in an area where your hand could not reach. You can order this tool on the Internet.

Whether you are using your hand or a tool, the same rules apply—gentle pressure and always toward comfort. It can be tempting to use a tool to apply deeper pressure and that is usually part of their design and use. Please remember, deep pressure and pain are not in harmony with this method. Be creative. You can also lean against a doorframe and shift your body slightly to put a tight muscle along your spine at rest. If it's your lower back, maybe a doorknob on a tender spot and shifting your body will work. Use extra caution and gentleness while using tools other than your hands, as you may not be immediately aware of the amount of pressure you are applying and may cause bruising, particularly if you are using blood thinners.

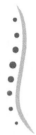

Chapter 5
WHAT YOU DON'T KNOW CAN HURT YOU!

"Air coming into the body does not cause the ribs and diaphragm to move—that's backwards. The lungs don't do anything by themselves—they depend upon surrounding structures (the ribs and diaphragm) to move. If it weren't for the ribs and diaphragm moving, the lungs would just sit there like a liver or an appendix."
– David Vining

My First Rib Is Where?
I never thought ribs could be somewhere other than where they belonged, until I had pleurisy. Pleurisy is an irritation to the lungs that makes breathing painful and involves a lot

49

of coughing. During a particularly difficult coughing spell, I felt something shift in my back by my shoulder blade and suddenly, every already painful breath now included a stabbing pain in my back. I called my chiropractor, who was able to help me correct the shifted rib, and I had immediate relief.

Ribs can shift for all kinds of reasons—falls, sports injuries, accidents (car and otherwise), falling off a horse, reaching, twisting, lifting (especially with arms extended), and upper back tension (especially along the spine and between the neck and shoulders). Of course, I knew generally where my ribs were, but I was surprised to find out how high they go. The first rib attaches just below the base of the neck in back and just under the collarbone in front. The upper ribs can be felt deep in the armpit. When the first rib is being pulled out of position by tension in the muscles of the upper back, it can be felt as a hard knot across the top of the shoulder area midway between the shoulder joint and the neck. In between the collar bone and the top of the shoulder blade it can become quite tender. That shift in position starts a negative spiral, because now the muscles must stand guard to stabilize the ribs that are out of position and no one in that whole neighborhood gets to be at home in their comfy chair!

In my experience, chronic mid and upper back pain and tension are nearly always related to one or more ribs shifted out of position. Some other occurrences of pain that result when ribs are not at home are the following:

1. Stabbing pain by the shoulder blade.

   (This is the most common description of middle and upper ribs that have shifted out of position, whether due to an impact or tension.)

2. Numbness or tingling in fingers.

   (Numbness and/or tingling can indicate nerves being compressed, which can occur at the neck, at any of the joints of the arm, or when the first rib is lifted by tension and presses against the collar bone, which can compress part of the nerve bundle going to the arm.)

3. Restriction or pain while breathing, especially deep breathing.

4. Tight muscles around the ribs.

   (The ribs cannot fully expand because of the tension, which also restricts the lungs, making it difficult to take a full breath. At times, this pain can be sharp and make it difficult to do daily tasks and get adequate sleep.)

5. Pain in the chest and shortness of breath.

    (These are classic heart attack symptoms and ribs out of position can also be described this way. I have had a few clients come in after getting a clean bill of health from their cardiologist with mysterious chest pain on the left side and difficulty taking a deep breath. Their symptoms resolved fully when ribs were released to go back home.)

6. Tender knots in the upper trapezius—the space between the neck and shoulder joint—that may come and go.

    (When the first rib is lifted by the upper trapezius muscle it can result in burning, tenderness, and/or pain across the line from the neck to the shoulder. When you put the upper trapezius muscle at rest it fills with blood and allows any of the top three ribs that have been pulled out of position to go back to their homes. This is described in chapter 6 as the Upper Trapezius Release.)

7. Pain in the armpit with or without a knot.

   (The upper ribs can be accessed deep in the armpit. Once I had a pain in my armpit that came up quickly. It felt quite tender so I did the muscle release technique for a few minutes and the knot and pain went away. It crossed my mind that it might be a swollen lymph node, which can be a cause for concern for an upper-body infection, but when it resolved effortlessly with no further pain, I let go of any worry.)

8. Difficulty in taking a deep breath and a feeling of tightness in the chest.

   (Some clients have said this sensation resembles asthma, but does not respond to an inhaler or asthma medication. It makes sense that the symptoms would not respond to medication because it is due to muscle tension restricting the rib cage and therefore the lungs.)

As with many other issues in life, prevention is easier than a cure when it comes to the toll of stress on the body. Overall life stress, as well as tension from sitting at a desk for long hours (possibly with poor posture), contact sports, twisting while lifting, prolonged coughing, and falls are effective recipes for rib trouble. Building a list of strategies that work for you to reduce your body's reaction to life stress will give you action steps to take when the pressure is on and thinking becomes challenging. Mindful breathing is a great item for the list, as it can alleviate stress and also provides mobility for your ribs. A simple definition of mindful breathing is paying attention to breath coming in and going out and the movement in your upper body as you breathe.

Homecoming

When it comes to ribs, my Mom's experience has been one of the most amazing rib stories to me. I had recently graduated from massage school and had been learning about releasing tight muscles and ribs while working full time as a massage therapist. For her eighty-first birthday, I took my massage table over and offered to release every tight muscle we could find. It took three hours. When I had her turn to lie on her back, she said, "Oh, I have always wondered if it's normal that my ribs on this side are higher than the ones on the other side," as she pointed toward the ceiling.

I responded that I wasn't willing to call her abnormal, but I was pretty sure she wasn't born that way! I started releasing the tight muscles restricting her rib cage. She lay on her opposite side and for the top four ribs, each one was more comfortable and released with a slightly backward and upward movement. It occurred to me that these ribs had probably all shifted at the same time on the same day from an impact to this entire side of her back. I decided to stretch my hands out to encompass the whole rib cage and go slightly backward and upward, which she reported to be very comfortable. Even though muscles usually fill with blood and release their tension when put at rest for twenty to forty-five seconds, I decided to hold the position for a whole minute since it seemed like it may have been a big deal when it happened. After doing a small circular motion with both of my hands to integrate the changes, I had her lie down on her back again—and now both sides of her rib cage were even. She said, "I just took the deepest breath ever!" We both were in awe over what had just happened.

When I asked how many years ago she thought the accident might have happened, she couldn't think of any accidents that impacted only one side of her body, so I suggested she just wait and the memory might come to her. Within a few minutes, she gasped and said, "I was ten years old and my Mom said not to swing on the rope swing because the rope was rotten." She thought the rope looked just fine. I think we all know which side she fell on. She also said that she had lain there for a long time trying to get her breath.

As I thought about it later, I remembered reading in a book by midwife Elizabeth Davis that a newborn baby only breathes after its chest is born, because the lungs can't expand until the ribs can expand. I believe that is why my Mom had the sensation of taking a very deep breath on the newly released side. So, it seems that her breathing had been restricted on that side for seventy-one years! It has been over a year, and my Mom tells me that the ribs are still in their easy chairs. There have been several other cases of long-term rib injuries that were easily released, so it seems there is no "statute of limitations" for timing on rib releasing.

I recommend that you set a time each month to do this easy self-check on your ribs because movement and breath can be quite restricted and painful if some ribs are shifted out of position. If it continues, the restriction may impact neighboring areas and contribute to tension headaches, lower back pain, and jaw pain.

There are twelve pairs of ribs, and the middle and upper ones are like bucket handles because they attach in the front and back to bone with cartilage. The exception is the bottom two on each side, which only attach on the back. The other end "floats," which gives them the name of floating ribs. (See the image below.) Whether a rib is bumped out of place by an impact or pulled out of place by tension, the action may have only touched one part of the rib, but because it is a solid structure, the entire path of the rib is affected. Anywhere along the path that feels tender or raised out of position is a good place to start putting it at rest. I find it easiest to have people check their own ribs out on the side of their body because it is easily reached by most people with either the thumb of the hand on the same side, or by reaching across the front with the fingers of the opposite hand.

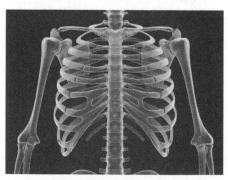

Fig. 6. X-ray showing rib positions

The rib release is very similar to the muscle release from chapter 4. Rereading the first section there can provide a quick review and you can check out the **"Rib Release Activity"** video on the website.

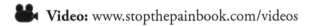 **Video:** www.stopthepainbook.com/videos

Note

A quick overview of the position of your ribs will be helpful before you do the specific check on your ribs. Place your thumbs deep in your armpits and lightly run them down the side of your body to your waist. Now do it again and notice the sensation of passing over hill, valley, hill, valley, etc. Now that you have some familiarity with the landscape, trace that path again while you notice whether you feel any of the hills (ribs) like a speed bump that is raised higher than its neighbors. Take note of that area to check carefully in the next phase. Now, starting under the bottom rib, press in on each rib lightly along the side of your body and pay attention to where you find tenderness or resistance to your pressure. You can make notes if you would like, but it is also fine to just release the tension around each rib that is out of position as you come to it.

Be Aware

If you have pain around specific ribs that is from a recent accident or injury, proceed very gently. If there is no relief after the first few rounds of very light touching on a particular rib, consider that your rib may be fractured and take appropriate action. If you choose to have an X-ray and a fracture is found, do not attempt to release the tight muscles until your care provider says the fracture is healed. In my experience with clients, time to heal is the only remedy that can be offered, if a fracture is found. When you hear of someone with fractured ribs and the care provider does nothing, it is helpful to know a little medical history before jumping to a conclusion of criticizing them for doing nothing. The old school remedy of binding the ribs was abandoned because bound ribs could not expand for breathing and the patient slowly suffocated. Breathing can be very painful when fractured ribs rise and fall, but that movement is essential.

Choose

Pick your right or left side to check first. You can use the thumb of your hand on the same side of your body or the first two fingers of your other hand and reach across your body. Picture a line from your hipbone at the side of your body to your armpit. Starting at your waist, begin pressing in along that line as you move upward a little at a time until you come to your bottom rib. If you found any tenderness between the waist and the bottom rib, make note of that to release by going toward comfort. The bottom two ribs on each side are only attached to the spine and are called floating ribs. Unless you have pain more toward the back in the area of the low ribs and want to check them specifically, you probably won't come in contact with them. Press in on the lowest rib along that imaginary line at the side of your body. When the muscles around the rib are not tight, the rib will have a slight springiness to it. You will feel the difference if you find any tight ribs—they will be like pushing against a small tree branch near the trunk rather than further out on the branch. Choose the first sore or restricted rib you come to.

Assess

Gently put two fingers on top of the sore or tender place and press in lightly to see what number on the pain scale you would give the discomfort. Make a note of it.

Determine

1. With two fingers placed lightly on the sore area, use just enough pressure to move the muscle a bit with your fingers without sliding your fingers along the skin or clothing.

2. Move your fingers forward or backward along the rib.

3. See which direction feels more comfortable and has more freedom of movement.

Release

Hold gently in the direction of comfort for twenty to forty-five seconds. Less tension requires less holding time, because the muscle is not as wrung out in terms of blood flow. Rib releases have an extra component—a special breathing technique that can be done while holding the rib in the release position if it doesn't respond fully the first time.

1. Take a medium breath, in through the nose and out through the mouth.

2. Take a deep, rib-expanding breath, and when you think your lungs are full, take in a little more and

hold it for a few seconds; then release slowly. You may feel a slight shift under your fingers as the rib returns to its comfy chair. Deep breathing can be seen as the body's natural physical therapy for ribs.

Integrate

At the end of the release move, make a few small circles with your fingers in either direction to integrate the changes. This action gets everyone in the neighborhood on the same page by telling them that the muscle you were working with has headed home and they can, too!

Check

See if the two opposite directions you checked before feel similar or balanced now, like both muscles are equally relaxed. If they are, one full cycle is complete. Areas with low to moderate tension may now be complete with every part home and in their comfy chair. By repeating the Assess step, you can determine whether there is still tenderness, suggesting you need to do another cycle.

Reassess

If you find no tenderness at the end of the first cycle, you can move up to the next rib. If the answer to the Assess step is "Yes," rate the remaining tenderness you found, and repeat the Release step.

Release

The spot may need one more round in the same direction, or it may be ready to release tension in the opposite direction. Your body will indicate what it needs; all you need to do is move the spot in the direction of ease and comfort. Go through the full cycle again, which takes less than a minute.

If there is still tension or tenderness at the end of the second cycle when you assess, try a small movement up or down across the rib. Repeat the cycle and assess. The diagonal directions that would form an X on the rib are the next steps. If you have released all eight compass directions and still find tenderness, the next step is to place two fingers on the tender spot again and hold the fingers together as you turn them slightly in a clockwise and then a counterclockwise direction. Again, if there is a difference, go in the direction of comfort and ease of movement. Hold for twenty to forty-five seconds, do the integrative circle, and recheck. If you still have tenderness, let the area rest for a few minutes while you release another tender spot along the same rib and come back to check it later.

The upper six ribs may also need to be released on the front (anterior) side, where they attach to the breastbone. Check both sides of the breastbone and use the compass directions to find comfort and release tension.

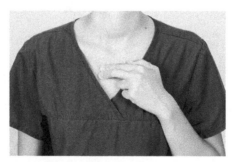

Fig. 7. Sample release position for upper ribs on front

The side of the upper ribs are found deep in the armpit. Tension can cause the upper trapezius muscle to lift the upper three ribs out of position. If you have tension or a burning sensation across the shoulders between the neck and the shoulder joint, go to chapter 6 and do the technique called "Shrug, Chicken Wing, Lean" to release the muscle tension so those ribs can go home. If there is still an issue with tenderness in the area of the upper ribs, try reaching along the spine in the upper back with the opposite arm from the front to reveal a tender area that needs release.

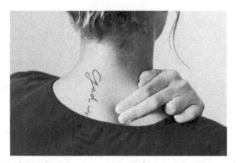

Fig. 8. Sample release position for upper ribs on back

When the top rib is lifted out of position, it can be felt as a tender knot between the neck and the shoulder joint in the space between the collar bone and the top of the shoulder blade. If it doesn't respond fully to the release in the arm pit and by the breastbone, check for tenderness along the collarbone and use the compass directions to release the tension from those tender spots. Movements will be very small with the collarbone, but release is very effective.

Often a client will say that a spot is much less tender and that we can move on. I know it is hard to imagine that the tenderness will go away completely, but typically it does when each rib is in its comfy chair. I encourage you to try another round or two when tenderness is slight to see if the last little step to get to the comfy chair can be taken care of right then. I'm glad for a person's attitude of gratitude for the area that is much better, and I encourage them to go beyond "tolerable recovery." Sure, you could live with a tiny bit of pain, but why not give each rib the chance to be totally home?

On a few occasions, I have seen two ribs that seemed to be too close together. To check rib spacing, I start at the bottom rib along the side of the body and touch each rib and the spaces between them. Normally, part of my finger pad will fit in the space between ribs. When there is strong tension in the small intercostal muscles between the ribs, my finger pad won't go in between the ribs much at all. The space is too small and the muscle too tight. The first thought is to want to spread them apart, but the tight muscles are very good at "stabilizing the situation" to protect you, so that won't work. The strategy is to lightly bring the two ribs that are too close together even closer together to release the tension and let the muscles fill with blood. After thirty seconds or so, the muscles are usually more pliable and will allow the ribs to move toward home. It may need one more squeeze motion to release fully. Remember, the rule of thumb is still *no pain, only comfort*, in the releasing process.

If trying to follow this process with words alone is difficult, the video will make it much clearer. I encourage you to watch the video and see how simple the cycle is with visual input and sound. In the unusual event that there is still a strong pain or other sensation after you have watched the video and released the rest of the area, feel free to email me your experiences or questions. If it is difficult to explain, we can arrange a video conference call to see if it would be helpful to work together. If you have not yet checked with a local healthcare provider, consider enlisting their help. I have seen this method work so well for so many people that I want to be sure that you have every opportunity to learn and implement it effectively for yourself.

The video that demonstrates this section is **"Rib Release Activity."**

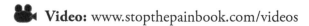 **Video:** www.stopthepainbook.com/videos

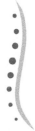

Chapter 6
COMFORT ZONE

"The doctor of the future will give no medication but will interest his patients in the care of the human frame, diet, and in the cause and prevention of disease."
– Thomas Edison

When we are focusing on pain in any area of life, it is characterized by tension, lack, and restriction. When we make a shift and focus on seeking comfort, the same area transforms into a place of release, flow, and abundance. The purpose of this chapter is to give a brief overview of some amazing and easy muscle release tools you can use in daily life to reduce stress and back or neck pain.

Release Your Core

I had the privilege of taking a course from Liz Koch, who has given her career to studying the psoas muscle, which is commonly seen as just a muscle that functions as a hip flexor and leg rotator. The psoas is one of the longest muscles in the body, connecting the low back to the legs, so it has a clear connection to low back pain. She has written extensively on its vital role as part of our core being, so I will refer you to her for details on its importance. Simple release techniques like Constructive Rest Position, found in chapter 6 of *The Psoas Book,* can be helpful when done for ten minutes once or twice a day. The following pictures show two versions of the Constructive Rest Position. The position with knees and hips bent at ninety-degree angles may be more comfortable if you have low back issues. The demonstration video is **"Release Your Core."**

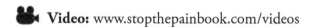 **Video:** www.stopthepainbook.com/videos

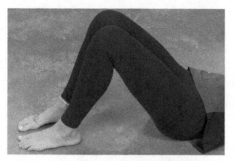

Fig. 9. Core release with feet on the floor

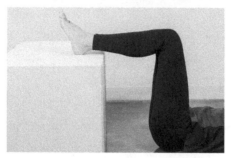

Fig. 10. Core release with hips and knees at ninety degrees

Another key takeaway I found from the course is related to posture. Our seating options today are soft, and the seats in our cars are bucket seats. Liz points out that the intended place for our weight to rest when we sit is not a circle around our buttocks, but the "sit bones" at the base of our pelvis. Try sitting on a firm chair, leaning against the back of the chair, and noticing how your back feels. Then, put a small folded towel under your sit bones or move out closer to the front of the chair so that your knees can be slightly lower than your hips and sit on your sit bones with your back away from the back of the chair. The result is often less strain in the upper back and better posture. When the hips round and roll backward, the shoulders tend to round forward. When the hips roll forward to put the sit bones in contact with the chair, the shoulders move back into a more natural position. Liz also suggests folding up a towel or finding a book of the right size to fill the "bucket" of your car seat to assist with effortless good posture while driving.

There is a surprising connection between the psoas and emotions, stress, trauma, and so on. This is the muscle that contracts to bring a baby into fetal position. In a situation that is perceived as threatening, even as adults, the psoas contracts involuntarily to attempt to pull the body into a "safe" position and it may remain contracted. The brain may get the message that, "Tight is the new normal." Daily activities like extended periods of sitting, excessive running/ walking, many sit-ups, sitting in a soft chair, or even sleeping in a fetal position can add to the strain on the psoas.

Dr. Christine Northrup has written an informative article called "Why Your Psoas Muscle Is the Most Vital Muscle in Your Body." Dr. Northrup's article summarizes some of Liz Koch's and others' materials, and she lists seven signals of a psoas imbalance: difference in leg length, knee and low back pain, postural problems, difficult bowel movements, menstrual cramps, chest breathing, and exhaustion. Several people commented on the article that TREs (trauma-releasing exercises) taught by Dr. Bercelli are very effective at releasing stuck emotions that impact the psoas. If you have mystery groin or abdominal pain that may affect your back or breathing, check into this little-known issue and these options for resetting your brain's definition of "normal" to one that is more relaxed and balanced.

Even though the psoas muscle is more commonly associated with the hip area, it is attached to the lower five vertebrae in the lumbar spine, so it is commonly involved in low back pain. A very helpful video for a pain free seated psoas release can be found with a YouTube search for "ortho-bionomy self care hip".

Forward Head Posture

For decades, a forward head position has been associated with aging, but due to increased time spent using cell phones, tablets and other handheld technology, an epidemic of forward head posture (FHP), "text neck," or "tech neck," has affected all ages, even young people. Rounded shoulders are a classic sign. Problems that can result are neck and shoulder pain, muscle spasms, muscle fatigue, headaches, poor posture, and TMJ (jaw) pain. To do a quick self-check, have someone take a side view, full-body picture with a phone or camera and stretch a string on the screen or print it out and draw a line from bottom to top through the middle of your ankle, knee, hip, and shoulder. If the middle of your ear is forward of the line, you have some degree of forward head posture. For each inch your head is forward of your shoulders, the effect is ten pounds of added pressure to your neck.

A helpful app and book/video set I've found is the 30-Day Posture Makeover by Michelle Joyce, which gives exercises and tips for good posture while standing, sitting, walking, driving, sleeping, and other daily activities. Her perspective is that healthy body positioning will lead to relaxed muscles and easily sustainable good posture.

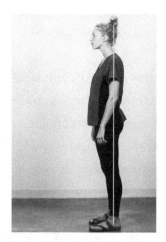

Fig. 11. Full-body picture for posture check

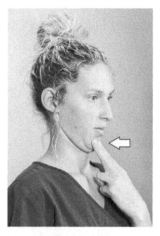

Fig. 12. Chin tuck exercise

One helpful exercise that is commonly recommended to combat forward head posture is the chin tuck. While standing with your back to a wall with your best posture, tuck your chin until you feel a slight stretch at the back of your neck. Once you know what this feels like, you can use the headrest in a car to lean against or just stand, sit, or lie and press on your chin. Five repetitions for five seconds each, several times a day, is a common recommendation. Another simple test is to stand with your back against a wall and see if your head naturally touches the wall with ease. If you need to press your head back to reach the wall or it feels tired after holding it against the wall for a minute, you may have FHP.

A friend who is a physiatrist sees patients daily who are in pain and she shared with me that she has seen an increase in pain and dysfunction related to handheld technology use. It was sobering to hear her say that she anticipates seeing the average age of her clients decreasing in the coming years until a large part of her practice will be helping young people with pain due to posture issues.

The January 2017 newsletter of Auspice Safety Inc. gives tips to reduce FHP: avoid using handheld technology for lengthy work, call using a headset rather than texting repeatedly, have the top third of your computer monitor at eye level, bring wireless devices to eye level, increase text size to avoid leaning toward your device, change positions every fifteen minutes or so, and do neck stretches and strengthening exercises frequently. The newsletter also recommends getting an ergonomic evaluation of your workspace to correct positions that may be contributing to muscle imbalances. Check with your spine health provider for a full assessment and an individualized correction program if you think you have an issue.

8 Steps to A Pain-Free Back: Natural Posture, authored by Esther Gokhale, is a helpful resource for reversing the negative effects of gravity on our posture. She traveled to places in the world where only 5 percent of the adult population had ever experienced back pain. Esther studied their movements, sitting habits, and standing postures and distilled it all down so that we can learn their secrets. I find it very encouraging that even back issues that we have come to think of as permanent, like a Dowager's hump in the upper back, can begin to resolve with purposeful movement. I'm planning to have better posture this year than I had in my younger years. Would you like to join me? See the demonstration video **"Forward Head Posture."**

 Video: www.stopthepainbook.com/videos

Upper Trapezius Release
(aka Shrug, Chicken Wing, Lean)

The upper trapezius muscle that reaches from your neck out to your shoulders is usually one of the muscles that feels the strain when we spend long hours at the computer or looking down at a device. When you feel a burning sensation across the top of the shoulders between the neck and the shoulder joint, this exercise provides a good release. You can see it demonstrated in the **"Shrug, Chicken Wing, Lean"** video.

📹 **Video:** www.stopthepainbook.com/videos

- Stand with the shoulder of the side you want to release first about twelve to eighteen inches from a wall. (You are standing with your shoulders perpendicular to the wall.)
- Shrug the shoulder nearest the wall so that your shoulder is near your ear.

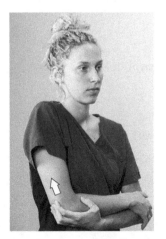

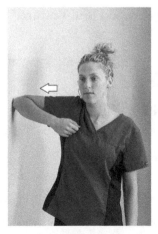

Fig. 13. Upper trapezius release start position

Fig. 14. Upper trapezius release finish position

- With your shoulder still shrugged up, lift your elbow toward the wall so that it is parallel to the floor (like a chicken wing).

- Lean into the wall.

- Hold this position for forty-five seconds and notice any warmth you may feel as blood comes into the upper trapezius muscle across the top of the shoulder to your neck.

- Bring your arm down and with the help of your other hand, circle your shoulder around gently. You want to use your other hand to assist in this motion so you don't immediately engage the muscle you just released.

- Bring your elbow back up to the chicken wing position and pull gently out to your side and in an arc forward on your elbow with the opposite hand to give a light traction to your shoulder area and open up space where it has been tight.

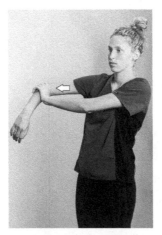

Fig. 15. Upper trapezius light traction start position

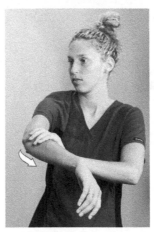

Fig. 16. Upper trapezius light traction finish position

Use Your Imagination

I encourage you to use a wide variety of strategies to bring relaxation to your body. You can imagine you are lying on a beach, in a mountain meadow, or anywhere you find peaceful. It may be a place you have enjoyed before or you can use your imagination and envision a new place every day! Turn on some relaxing music and take a "staycation."

Breathing

Since breathing is one of the activities of the body that is automatic, we can be grateful that it's not required to notice your breathing in order to stay alive! Your mind and body already know what to do in case of an emergency. If you were being chased by a bear, your body would increase your rate of breathing and heart rate to provide what you would need to run away from it or fight it off. In an emergency, whether real or perceived, you are fully present in that very moment and your body is in survival mode. If your heart is racing from an emergency message like an unexpected bill, an argument, difficulty in traffic, or a deadline, you can encourage your pulse rate to return to normal by consciously slowing your breathing down and noticing the air as it flows into and out of your body. When you are consciously controlling the breathing process and slowing the breath rate, it helps your brain to understand that the environment is safe now and the bear is evidently gone because your breathing is now in safe mode. Muscle tension is also releasing at that point.

Regarding breathing, Liz Koch teaches in *The Psoas Book* about the tension and restriction created when the fear response is active in the body. She suggests that breathing is better when *released* into its natural flow than trained into an artificial, regimented pattern. On an internal level, if I am concerned about "getting it right" with regard to breathing, I am setting myself up for comparing myself, being judgmental toward myself, and creating an atmosphere of restriction instead of acceptance and release. A friend explained that his type of personality benefitted from using a very structured method of breath training to explore the scope of possibilities with breath and now he is more proficient and ready to discover his personal breathing patterns for different situations. You may already be confident that you can develop your natural flow of breathing or you may choose to find a supportive method that encourages your breath to be natural, free, and unrestricted. I encourage you to trust yourself and believe that you are the best one to recognize what works well for you. We each get to have our own journey to find release and an easy flow of breath.

If you look for instructions on breathing techniques, I recommend that you look for one that includes both the diaphragm and upper chest. In order for the lungs to fill completely, the diaphragm must contract downward to pull air into the bottom of the lungs. Also, the upper ribs and chest must expand up and out so that the upper portion of the lungs can fully expand to bring air in. As you gain familiarity and proficiency with the movements of the chest and abdomen in full chest and lung expansion, your breathing will become natural and flowing and will not require conscious thought.

One of my favorite relaxation techniques is to tune in and pay attention to five breaths. With each breath in, notice how the breath comes into the abdominal area. With each exhale, let the body relax progressively. Sometimes I will relax the head and neck with the first breath, then move down the body with each breath. By the last breath, I am often feeling limp, like the tension has drained out. Sharing the experience with a loved one can increase the peace even further!

Prayer/Meditation/Mindfulness

These activities can lower blood pressure and increase relaxation in the body on many levels, including a calmer brainwave pattern. The positive benefits of these practices carry forward as you go on with your day. There are many apps that can help you develop healthful habits of being mindful and meditating.

Neck Release

Tension in the neck muscles that is stronger on one side than the other can tug one or more neck vertebrae off toward that side. An easy way to detect this shift is to place the fingers of each hand vertically along the sides of the neck, starting at the base of the skull. Gently move the fingers down to the base of the neck, noticing the position of each vertebra in relation to its neighbors. When they are well aligned, they will be directly on top of each other like marbles in a skinny tube sock.

If you feel one shifted slightly to one side, place a finger on each side to gently exaggerate the pattern further to that side to make the tight muscle slack so that it can fill with blood. It is a small movement and should not hurt. Hold for 20-45 seconds (or you can count 3 breaths) and move the area in a small circle a few times with your fingers to integrate the changes. Then recheck. Usually, the vertebrae will be more centered and the area will be less tense. You can repeat again or move in a slightly different direction to release further tension and restore movement and function more fully.

I also like to draw infinity loops (horizontal figure eights) in the air with my nose to relax my neck. I start by looking straight ahead. To release higher on my neck, I tip my head up a little higher and continue drawing infinity loops. The uppermost neck joint is mobilized when looking toward the ceiling; the lowest, when looking toward the floor. The video **"Neck Release Figure Eights"** will make this easy to understand.

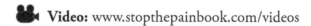 **Video:** www.stopthepainbook.com/videos

Isometric Exercises

These exercises have a dual benefit—they can strengthen muscles and release tension. The neck has three axes of movement and each has a corresponding isometric release. Each release movement can be done twice in a row with added benefit and it can be done several times a day. If you check your range of motion first, you can appreciate seeing the benefits after you do the muscle release techniques.

The first movement is taking your ear toward your shoulder. See how far your head can easily lean to the left by moving your head so that your ear moves toward your left shoulder. Now bring your head back to neutral position and lower your right ear toward your right shoulder.

Release: See Fig. 17 and Fig. 18 for start and finish positions. From the position shown, press your head lightly into your hand for five to ten seconds, then release the effort and use either hand to gently bring the head to follow

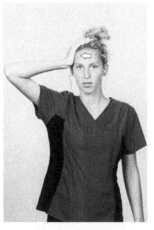

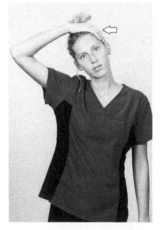

Fig. 17. Ear to shoulder isometric release start position

Fig. 18. Ear to shoulder isometric release finish position

through in the direction of motion you were pressing to end in the finish position shown. Always stay within the comfort range during the isometric press and follow-through motion.

Next, turn to look out across shoulder. See how far your head can easily turn to the left as if you were turning to look behind you. Now bring your head back to neutral position and see how far you can easily turn toward your right shoulder.

Release: See Fig. 19 and Fig. 20 for start and finish positions. From the position shown, press your head lightly into your hand for five to ten seconds, then release the

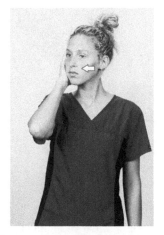

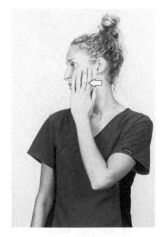

Fig. 19. Looking back isometric release start position

Fig. 20 Looking back isometric release finish position

effort and use either hand to gently bring the head to follow through in the direction of motion you were pressing to end in the finish position shown. Always stay within the comfort range during the isometric press and follow-through motion.

The final motion is taking your ear toward your shoulder, then looking up and back. See how far your head can easily lean to the left by moving your head so that your ear moves toward your left shoulder, then look up and back. Now bring your head back to neutral position and lower your right ear toward your right shoulder and look up and back.

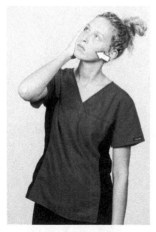

Fig. 21. Ear to shoulder plus look back isometric release start position

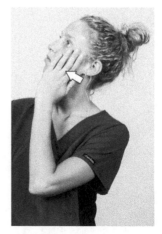

Fig. 22. Ear to shoulder plus look back isometric release finish position

Release: See Fig. 21 and Fig. 22 for start and finish positions. From the position shown, press your head lightly into your hand for five to ten seconds, then release the effort and use either hand to gently bring the head to follow through in the direction of motion you were pressing to end in the finish position shown. Always stay within the comfort range during the isometric press and follow-through motion.

 Video: www.stopthepainbook.com/videos

Spindle Cell Technique

Spindle cells in the muscles are part of the proprioceptive system in the body. Simply put, they tell your body where it is in space by providing feedback to the nerves and brain about the amount of tension in the muscle and how fast it is changing. They make it possible for you to reach something you know is behind you without turning around because your body knows exactly where your hand is, even without input from your eyes. I learned this concept in Touch for Health classes with instructors Deb Jenkins and Larry Green.

The spindle cell technique is very powerful for releasing tension, as it can reset the brain's relationship with the muscle. Under some circumstances, when a muscle contracts, the brain gets the message that tight is the new normal. To reset it, start near the center of the tight muscle and take your thumb and first finger and make a "pinching" motion a few times that includes the skin and the muscle layers just below it. Now recheck the tension. Alternatively, if it is in an area you can easily reach with both thumbs, you can push your thumbs toward each other near the belly or center of the tight muscle a few times. This motion communicates to the brain that the parts of the spindle cells are too close together and the brain needs to give the signal to reduce the tension. Recheck muscle tension and repeat as needed.

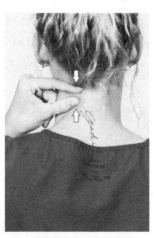

Fig. 23. Spindle cell release

If you have a muscle that has the opposite issue and needs to be toned up because it has become flaccid or lax, reversing the motion will send the message that the spindle cells of the muscle are too far apart and need to be brought together or contracted by signals from the brain. Place your thumbs together in the belly of the muscle and stroke away from the center a few times to prompt the brain to reset and contract the muscle fibers. The video **"Spindle Cell Technique"** will make this quick and powerful technique clear.

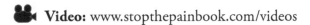 **Video:** www.stopthepainbook.com/videos

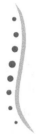

Chapter 7

MOVING FORWARD

"Physical well-being necessitates listening to what you already know, and then taking it seriously enough to act accordingly. When you wake up and feel the impulse to arch your back, stretch, and exhale with a loud sigh,… do it."

– Darrell Caulkins

Will This Relief Last?

If the members of your body have gone home and are not being pushed or pulled back out of their homes, they are very happy to remain home. For pain that stems from repetitive motions (think of the work done by hairdressers, dental professionals, computer users, etc.), it is important to learn the appropriate ways to move the muscles involved in the repetitive movement so that they won't create strain on the body. Proper body mechanics and sitting or standing positions are key. Taking a body awareness class like the Alexander technique or Feldenkrais may help you refine your movement patterns. Adapting your environment (i.e., chair or desk height), and selecting suitable ergonomic equipment could save you from pain and healthcare expenses down the road. As the ergonomics field expands, more practitioners are becoming available to give individualized help to tailor your environment to your needs. Another key concept is to provide frequent breaks during repetitive motions, even if it just a few seconds to move the area around every few minutes and a few minutes every half hour to an hour.

Questions + Listening = Helpful Answers

If parts of your body seem to not be staying in their homes, try being curious and asking questions, then writing down insights that come to you to help you see patterns.

Ask the following questions regarding pain:

- When do I notice the pain?
- Does anything relieve it?
- What aggravates it?
- When did it start? If the origin isn't clear, try asking these questions:
    o When do I remember not having this pain? (How long ago?)
    o When do I first remember noticing it?
    o What was happening in my life between those two times?

Ask the following questions regarding stress and tension:

- What would help me release tension right now? Ideas: exercise, a warm bath, herbal tea, walking barefoot outside, sunshine time, closing my eyes and focusing on my breathing
- What stressor could I reduce or remove from my life this week? Ideas: leave for work fifteen minutes earlier to avoid some traffic, pack a lunch the night before to feel less rushed, draw a boundary in a toxic relationship, limit exposure to negative news

- What would bring me comfort right now? Ideas: a warm blanket, peaceful music, remembering a good time with a friend, reading a favorite piece of literature out loud
- What muscles could I strengthen to reduce physical stress? Get insight from a chiropractor, physical therapist, personal trainer, or other professional if you are not familiar with the big picture of movement, muscle interactions, and muscle balance.

When we need to establish self-care routines for getting out and staying out of pain, getting in touch with our deep motivation can be a key to lasting changes. If your reason for getting out of pain isn't immediately apparent or a previous motivator isn't relevant right now, sit and listen to your heart as you ask questions like these:

- What activity do I miss or want to learn?
- Where would I like to travel and what physical activity would I like to do there?
- What joyful activity would I like to be able to experience with someone I love?

- Do I want to be able to get back to work or start a new vocation?
- What emotional or spiritual value would I like to increase?
- In what way would I like to increase my knowledge or memory?

Regarding self-care

Self-care and self-compassion are more important than words can express. When this care is continually compromised, the stage is set for chronic tension and pain to build up eventually. Today, care may look like taking more frequent breaks during work, asking for assistance rather than moving something heavy alone, getting a massage, or selecting water to drink with lunch. Your list will be unique to you. If it is difficult to think of what might be rejuvenating for you, try thinking of ten nice things you might do to show care for a friend and then do some of them for yourself—or with the friend! Choosing to ask, listen to, and trust your body and your intuitive sense of what would be best for you in every area of your life will bring you to answers you can live with.

I find that life works better if I communicate my needs rather than hoping someone else will read my mind. It is important to ask yourself whether you are exercising your power and taking responsibility for your results, or have you handed responsibility off to someone else and then gotten frustrated because you don't like the consequences. Reading this book and applying what you find comfortable is an example of taking responsibility for and honoring your wellbeing.

Dr. Caroline Leaf has written a book I find very interesting with recommendations for health and happiness called *Switch On Your Brain: The Key to Peak Happiness, Thinking, and Health.* As I grow in willingness to care for myself, I keep finding and implementing new ideas that are adding up to better health on several levels. Perhaps you can find a like-minded friend and enjoy the journey together.

Regarding sleep

Issues with sleep are important to resolve, as restorative sleep is a key for each of your body systems and overall health. The National Sleep Foundation reports that pain, stress, and poor health are the main issues that negatively affect sleep duration and quality. Chronic pain sufferers generally have a higher incidence of sleep problems impacting their daily lives. They feel less in control of their sleep and report being more sensitive to noise, light, temperature, and mattress comfort. Taking steps to reduce these challenges can help.

Putting a priority on getting sleep correlates with lengthier and better quality sleep, even for those with pain issues. Each additional night of compromised sleep can feed worry about the next night. As your pain decreases with using the strategies you have learned, I encourage you to dare to believe that your sleep will improve and get better nightly. I also recommend that you decide in advance to not let a night or two of less sleep trigger the worry cycle.

If sleep is difficult, you might try some of the following ideas:

- Take a warm bath before bed.
- Adding Epsom salt increases magnesium levels, which promotes relaxation.
- Add pillows for joint support.
- For side sleeping, a pillow that extends from the knees down to the ankles can support the low back, hips, knees, and ankles. Putting a supporting pillow only at the knees can create a strained position for the knee of the upper leg.

- Add a pillow that supports your neck and keeps the neck in line with the spine.
- If you aren't sure how to place pillows, try researching "sleep posture" to get ideas. If you wake up in pain that leaves as you get up and move around, it might be a problem with the mattress or sleep position more than your back.
- Diffuse essential oils to promote sleep.
- Lavender is popular and some studies suggest that a blend of oils created for sleep is more helpful than a single essential oil.
- Reduce sensitivity to light by wearing an eye mask.
- Use a noise machine or ear plugs to reduce the effect of sleep disturbing noises in the night.
- Expose yourself to bright light during the day to help regulate your sleep/wake cycle.
- Establish a sleeping/waking routine.
- The field of study called sleep hygiene offers several helpful ideas.
- Avoid caffeine and alcohol late in the day.
- Limit stimulating blue light exposure from electronic devices two hours before bedtime.

Your device may have settings to reduce blue light after a certain time automatically, or you can download an app to assist you. There are also glasses that block blue light from electronics.

- Relax and clear your mind in the evening.
- Listen to soothing music to set the tone for sleep.
- Get some exercise during the day that doesn't aggravate pain—though not right before bed.
  Explore isometric exercises, as they do not require much movement, but still add strength.
- Establish a reminder to go to the bathroom right before lying down and reduce your intake of liquids one to two hours before bed to avoid having to wake in the night.
- Try an app to help identify sleep patterns.
  I use Sleep Cycle, which uses the phone's microphone to identify activity levels and depth of sleep. I can add sleep notes about activities during the day and other factors that might impact sleep, then the software builds graphs to show the results. I prefer to put my phone on airplane mode to limit EMF exposure since it is only a few feet away from me.

- See a sleep doctor.

  A sleep specialist may be a good choice if you don't find solutions after trying some of these ideas. If you have sleep apnea, a sleep study can give you valuable information about oxygen levels and sleep interruptions.

Add your own notes to this list as you find things that work for you. Others around you may appreciate hearing what is helping your sleep patterns. I have been surprised at the number of people I know who talk about having ongoing issues with sleep once I start the conversation.

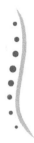

CONCLUSION

I hope this book has encouraged you to listen to your body. I believe that you can trust that you will know what your body is saying and that you can respond to what it needs. Keep learning, sharing, and doing. One of the best ways to learn a new activity is to share it.

I recommend making a list of 10 stress busters that work for you. You can do an Internet search to see what other people have found helpful or ask friends if you need a few more suggestions. Try out new ideas and see what feels supportive to you. Then, each day choose any three to enjoy. It can add up to make a big difference.

Take Some Time to Dream

Ask yourself, "What will I do when this pain isn't limiting me anymore? Remember that getting to comfort and staying there may be a process of tweaking your activities and posture, among other things, so you don't keep creating tension or making movements that push or pull things out of place. Keep moving forward. If you can get and sustain even 10 percent more comfort each week, you will be in a much better place sooner than you could have imagined.

Build comfort time into your schedule. You are worth it. Chances are, if you won't do it for yourself, no one else can do it for you.

I bless you with peace for your journey!

FURTHER READING

Gokhale, Esther, 8 *Steps to A Pain-Free Back: Natural Posture*, Pendo Press, 2008

Hansen, Fawne, *The Adrenal Fatigue Solution*, ebook

Koch, Liz, *Core Awareness*, North Atlantic Books, 2012

Koch, Liz, *The Psoas Book, Guinea Pig Publications, 2012*

Leaf, Caroline, *Switch On Your Brain: The Key to Peak Happiness, Thinking, and Health*, Baker Books, 2013

Olderman, Rick, *Fixing You: Back Pain, Boone Publishing, 2015*

Overmyer, Luann, *Ortho-Bionomy: A Path to Self-Care, North Atlantic Books, 2009*

Robin, Michelle, *Small Changes Big Shifts*, 2017

Sheppard, Jacquelyn, *Silent Takeover: How the Body Hijacks the Mind*, Destiny Image, 2016

ACKNOWLEDGEMENTS

Growing up with Dunham and Fenton roots meant there was always enough resourcefulness and resilience to solve the challenge at hand. Thanks, Mom and Dad, Jackie, Clint, John, your families, and all those who came before, for contributing to our "special sauce."

I'm grateful for my amazing children Josiah, Lydia, Jubilee, and Benjamin who have helped make each day a new adventure! I'm watching with joy as your journeys unfold and I'm cheering you on as you explore your unique contributions to the world.

Dawsyn, I love you and I'm so glad you were born! You bring joy to our lives every day. I encourage you to always be you, because everybody else is taken! I never knew how much love my heart could hold till you called me Nana.

Beverly launched me on my journey into bodywork, which led to getting my massage therapy license. The team at Massage Envy South in Olathe, Kansas, and my clients have given me so much. Dr. Tess introduced me to Ortho-Bionomy and Dr. Gayle helped me prepare for my massage therapy test. Linda loaned me confidence until I found my own as we worked together. Tiffany patiently held up a mirror showing me new ways of looking at life and how I respond to it. Deb and Larry have opened a whole new world to me with Touch for Health and other related training. Working with Dr. Robin and the supportive team at Your Wellness Connection is a dream come true. Thanks to all of you!

Hundreds of friends have contributed threads to the tapestry of me, and I'm forever grateful! We've worked, prayed, laughed, cried, and shared life together in Manhattan, Kansas, the Kansas City area, Kenya, Dallas, Colorado Springs, Winnipeg, and back to Kansas.

I don't want to leave anyone out, so I hesitate to start naming. I want to thank the current group of friends who have helped with this book journey over the past several months: Susan, Marge, Lydia, Jubilee, Terra, Cheryl, LaVerne, Pam, Ronda, Ashton, Suzanne, Linda, Jackie, Jenny, Eric, Jenn, Pat, Nathanael, Jordan, and Patrick. A special thanks to Phil and Linda, who have been there for me from the day I decided to write until the day I turned in the manuscript. Thank you for letting me hibernate in your little author tabernacle when I needed to focus on writing!

I am forever grateful to Dr. Angela Lauria and the team for coaching me and believing in me! You specialize in transformation that ripples out to the whole world. Thank you Todd Hunter and Trevor McCray for your help to bring my message forward. It's a privilege to make this journey with all of the other authors who bring such passion and commitment to their messages. You inspire me—thank you!

Words only begin to describe my gratitude to the Lord, who created me and encourages me forward. He said his name is "I AM…" and finishes the sentence in new ways each day with exactly what He knows I need. It's amazing to be fully known *and* fully loved. He wrote the book on transformation, and I'm glad to be his work of art (in progress)!

To the Morgan James Publishing team: Special thanks to David Hancock, CEO & Founder for believing in me and my message. To my Author Relations Manager, Margo Toulouse, thanks for making the process seamless and easy. Many more thanks to everyone else, but especially Jim Howard, Bethany Marshall, and Nickcole Watkins.

THANK YOU

As a thank you gift to you for getting my book, I would love to share with you a bonus video: **"Releasing TMJ Tension"** on the website below.

I would also like to get to know you and would love to jump on a call to customize your learning from the book, to find out if you chose this book for you or a loved one, and to REALLY hear YOUR story! Go ahead and grab a free 30-minute call time from my scheduler: calendly.com/stopthepainbook.

I look forward to chatting with you soon and helping you stop the pain now!

🎥 **Video:** www.stopthepainbook.com/videos

ABOUT THE AUTHOR

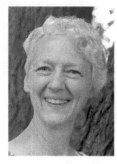 Vienna Dunham Schmidt has been helping people Stop the Pain with the gift in her hands since she was a teenager. In 2017 she entered the field of bodywork full-time after getting her massage therapy license. Vienna loves to see the look of hope and joy on her client's faces when they realize their brain has reset from "pain and tension are normal" to "comfort and ease are normal" by using simple pain-free methods. What she loves even more is when they step up to be the hero in their own journey out of pain and into comfortability. Vienna wrote Stop the Pain: Your Hands-on Manual for Neck and Back Relief to transfer that power into *your hands*!

Website: stopthepainbook.com

Email: vienna@stopthepainbook.com

Facebook: Stop the Pain Book

Printed in the USA
CPSIA information can be obtained
at www.ICGtesting.com
JSHW082358140824
68134JS00020B/2140

9 781642 796766